EA TOASTER OVEN AIR FRYER
RECIPE BOOK

Effective, Convenient and Affordable
Recipes for Faster, Wholesome and
Flavorful Meals that Anyone can Cook

Nancy M. Jack

Table of Contents

21. Teriyaki Pork Rolls

22. Rustic Pork Ribs

23. Ginger, Garlic And Pork Dumplings

24. Caramelized Pork Shoulder

25. Curry Pork Roast in Coconut Sauce

26. Chinese Salt and Pepper Pork Chop Stir-fry

27. Roasted Pork Tenderloin

28. Garlic Putter Pork Chops

29. Fried Pork with Sweet and Sour Glaze

30. Oregano-Paprika on Breaded Pork

31. Bacon Wrapped Pork Tenderloin

32. Dijon Garlic Pork Tenderloin

33. Pork Neck with Salad

34. Cajun Pork Steaks

35. Cajun Sweet-Sour Grilled Pork

36. Chinese Braised Pork Belly

37. Air Fryer Sweet and Sour Pork

38. Pork Loin with Potatoes

39. Fried Pork Scotch Egg

40. Roasted Char Siew (Pork Butt)

41. Juicy Pork Ribs Ole

42. Asian Pork Chops

CONCLUSION

INTRODUCTION

With a revolutionary kitchen appliance like the air fryer, cooking easy, healthy and delicious meals at home has become more practical. Not only will you be saving time but more importantly, you'll be cutting back on oil in your food.

What is an air fryer?

Before we move on, you might be wondering what an air fryer is exactly. Having made its debut in 2010, the air fryer is basically a kitchen appliance that fries without oil. Or, if need be, as little oil as possible. It does this by circulating hot air quickly with a built-in fan, a process that builds temperatures high enough to mimic conventional frying. Because of this, air fryers are able to fry food without the hazards of traditional oil frying – such as oil burns or fire damage – and can do it in a more systematic, controlled manner.

Functional principles

Since an air fryer uses hot air, some may argue that it works the same as a conventional oven. One, however, must remember that the two appliances produce different results, often due to their differences in technology. While ovens apply the dry air and heat directly onto the dish and take longer cooking times, air fryers contain a technology that rapidly spirals air around the dish, resulting in faster cooking times and a more fried appearance.

How to use an Air Fryer

Since 2010, there have been countless versions of the air fryer, often with different styles and mechanisms. That said, it's usually best to consult your service provider when it comes to how to use it, and if you're looking to replace your current brand with another, how it differs from your newer appliance. There are, however, some similarities:

Use the right attachment. Before anything else, clarify with the recipe what attachment you'll be needing for the dish. Do you need a mixer? A grill? And extra pan? Ensure that you have everything ready.

Unstick your pan. While air fryers don't need oil to work, not using oil often means a larger chance of certain dishes sticking to the pan or basket. That said, you can either mist the pan lightly with oil to keep your food from sticking or add parchment paper to it for a true oil-free alternative. Nonetheless, unsticking your pan is crucial.

Set the temperature. Whether you're using Fahrenheit, Celsius, or amount of wattage, be sure you set your fryer at the right temperature or power level so it doesn't over or undercook your dish. Some air fryers also provide "modes," or cooking options, for certain types of food like fries and pastries.

Set the timer. Once you're done with your temperature, just set the timer as indicated in the recipe and let it fly. You can experiment a little with this. Also, you can also take out the pan every now and then to add more ingredients or to check your cooking; all you need is to pause the machine.

Why use an air fryer?

First and foremost, the air fryer became popular for its numerous health benefits. The convenience and ease of use area close second and this combination make it an easy choice for those who want a healthy, delicious meal in a fraction of the time. For those who doubt the air fryer capabilities and prefer conventional cooking methods, perhaps the following points will be enough to convince them to make the switch to efficient cooking

A massive reduction in oil – no more than a tsp or two of foil is needed to cook food in an air fryer and yet it still achieves the same texture. A far cry from the many cups of oil that you would have to use to cook food in a deep fryer. The result is food that is not soaked in unhealthy fat that will clog the arteries

Easy press-and-go operation – No longer do you need to watch over your frying pan on your stove while frying your food. This also means no splattering of oil and accidental burns. All of the magic happens in the cooking chamber, just set your cooking preferences, push the right button, and let the air fryer do all of the work.

Bursting with flavor – the flavor of the food truly comes out in an air fryer. Despite the small amount of oil used in "frying" the food, the "fried" taste and texture is achieved

Cleaning made Easy – With food baskets that are dishwasher safe, it's as simple as removing it and putting it in. The cooking chamber can easily be cleaned with a cloth and a mild dishwashing soap

Safe – Its components are food safe and the cooking process itself helps you avoid kitchen accidents that can result in oil burns. The body of the air fryer hardly gets hot even if the temperature inside is at its highest. Using your standard kitchen gloves will give you more than enough protection when handling this kitchen appliance

Versatile unmatched – this modern appliance is more than just a fryer. You can bake, grill, and broil in it too. More of a highly versatile, mini convection oven rather than a fryer

Rapid cooking times – The high temperatures that are circulated in the cooking chamber cut common cooking times in half. This is because the heat is maintained throughout the time being cooked meaning you do not have to worry about the loss of heat slowing down your cooking

These benefits make air fryers the obvious choice when it comes to healthy cooking No compromise on flavor or convenience!

1. <u>Chicken Sausage Frittata with Cheese</u>

Preparation Time: 15 minutes

Cooking Time: 11 minutes

Servings: 2

INGREDIENTS

- 1 tablespoon olive oil
- 2 chicken sausages, sliced
- 4 eggs
- 1 garlic clove, minced
- 1/2 yellow onion, chopped
- Sea salt and ground black pepper, to taste
- 4 tablespoons Monterey-Jack cheese
- 1 tablespoon fresh parsley leaves, chopped

DIRECTIONS

1. Grease the sides and bottom of a baking pan with olive oil.
2. Add the sausages and cook in the preheated Air Fryer at 360 degrees F for 4 to 5 minutes.
3. In a mixing dish, whisk the eggs with garlic and onion. Season with salt and black pepper.
4. Pour the mixture over sausages. Top with cheese. Cook in the preheated Air Fryer at 360 degrees F for another 6 minutes.
5. Serve immediately with fresh parsley leaves. Bon appétit!

NUTRITIONS: 475 Calories 34.2g Fat 3g Carbs 36.2g Protein 2.6g Sugars

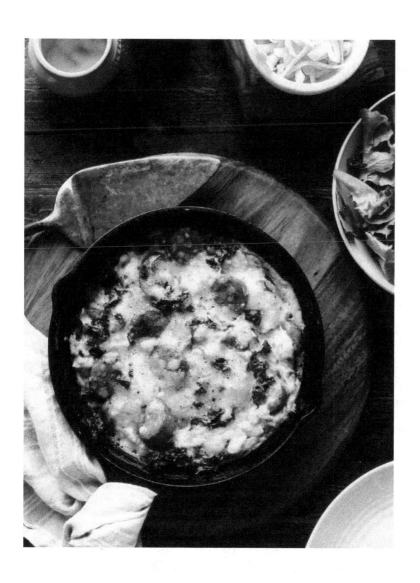

2. Traditional Chicken Teriyaki

Preparation Time: 50 minutes

Cooking Time: 18 minutes

Servings: 4

INGREDIENTS

- 1 ½ pounds chicken breast, halved
- 1 tablespoon lemon juice
- 2 tablespoons Mirin
- 1/4 cup milk
- 2 tablespoons soy sauce
- 1 tablespoon olive oil
- 1 teaspoon ginger, peeled and grated
- 2 garlic cloves, minced
- 1/2 teaspoon salt
- 1/2 teaspoon ground black pepper
- 1 teaspoon cornstarch

DIRECTIONS

1. In a large ceramic dish, place the chicken, lemon juice, Mirin, milk, soy sauce, olive oil, ginger, and garlic. Let it marinate for 30 minutes in your refrigerator.
2. Spritz the sides and bottom of the cooking basket with a nonstick cooking spray. Arrange the chicken in the cooking basket and cook at 370 degrees F for 10 minutes.

3. Turn over the chicken, baste with the reserved marinade and cook for 4 minutes longer. Taste for doneness, season with salt and pepper, and reserve.

4. Mix the cornstarch with 1 tablespoon of water. Add the marinade to the preheated skillet over medium heat; cook for 3 to 4 minutes. Now, stir in the cornstarch slurry and cook until the sauce thickens.

5. Spoon the sauce over the reserved chicken and serve immediately.

NUTRITIONS:

362 Calories

21.1g Fat

4.4g Carbs

36.6g Protein

2.4g Sugars

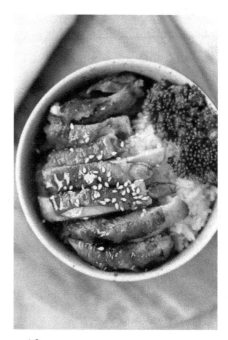

3. Loaded Chicken Burgers

Preparation Time: 30 minutes

Cooking Time: 12 minutes

Servings: 5

INGREDIENTS

- 2 tablespoons olive oil
- 1 onion, finely chopped
- 2 green garlic, chopped
- 6 ounces mushrooms, chopped
- 1 ½ pounds ground chicken
- 1/3 cup parmesan cheese
- 1/4 cup pork rinds, crushed
- 1 tablespoon fish sauce
- 1 tablespoon tamari sauce
- 1 teaspoon Dijon mustard
- 5 soft hamburger buns
- 5 lettuce leaves

DIRECTIONS

1. Heat a nonstick skillet over medium-high heat; add olive oil. Once hot, sauté the onion until tender and translucent, about 3 minutes.
2. Add the garlic and mushrooms and cook an additional 2 minutes, stirring frequently.
3. Add the ground chicken, cheese, pork rind, fish sauce, and tamari sauce; mix until everything is well incorporated.
4. Form the mixture into 5 patties. Transfer the patties to the lightly greased cooking basket.

5. Cook in the preheated Air Fryer at 370 degrees F for 8 minutes; then, flip them over and cook for 8 minutes on the other side.

6. Serve on burger buns, garnished with mustard and lettuce. Bon appétit!

NUTRITIONS: 476 Calories 29g Fa 29.9g Carbs 31.7g Protein 2.5g Sugars

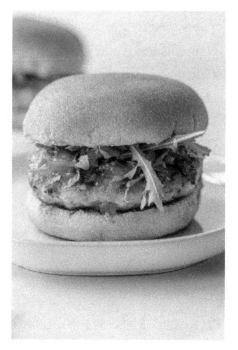

4. <u>Breaded Chicken Tenderloins</u>

Preparation Time: 15 minutes

Cooking Time: 15 minutes

Servings: 4

INGREDIENTS

- 1 egg, beaten
- 2 tablespoons vegetable oil
- ½ cup breadcrumbs
- 8 skinless, boneless chicken tenderloins

DIRECTIONS

1. In a shallow dish, beat the egg.
2. In another dish, add the oil and breadcrumbs and mix until a crumbly mixture forms.
3. Dip the chicken tenderloins into beaten egg and then coat with the breadcrumbs mixture.
4. Shake off the excess coating.
5. Set the temperature of Air Fryer to 355 degrees F. Grease an Air Fryer basket.
6. Arrange chicken tenderloins into the prepared Air Fryer basket in a single layer.
7. Air Fry for about 12-15 minutes.
8. Remove from Air Fryer and transfer the chicken thighs onto a serving platter.
9. Serve hot.

NUTRITIONS: Calories: 271 Carbohydrate: 12g Protein: 30.4g Fat: 11.5g Sugar: 0.9g Sodium: 113mg Pork Air Fry Recipes

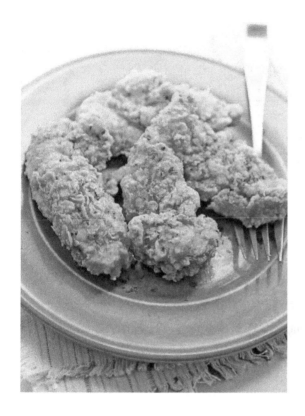

5.   <u>Saucy Pork Mince</u>

Preparation Time: 10 minutes

Cooking Time: 60 minutes

Serving: 8

INGREDIENTS

- 2 tablespoons olive oil
- 1 large onion, diced
- 2 lbs. ground pork
- 2 teaspoons salt

- 6 cloves garlic, chopped
- 1/2 cup red wine
- 6 cloves garlic, chopped
- 3 teaspoons ground cinnamon
- 2 teaspoons ground cumin
- 2 teaspoons dried oregano
- 1 teaspoon black pepper
- 1 can 28 oz. crushed tomatoes
- 1 tablespoon tomato passata

DIRECTIONS

1. Put a suitable wok over moderate heat and add oil to heat.
2. Toss in onion, salt, and pork meat then stir cook for 12 minutes.
3. Stir in red wine and cook for 2 minutes.
4. Add cinnamon, garlic, oregano, cumin, and pepper, then stir cook for 2 minutes.
5. Add tomato passata and tomatoes and cook for 20 minutes on a simmer.
6. Spread this mixture in a casserole dish.
7. Press "Power Button" of Air Fry Oven and turn the dial to select the "Bake" mode.
8. Press the Time button and again turn the dial to set the cooking time to 20 minutes.
9. Now push the Temp button and rotate the dial to set the temperature at 350 degrees F.
10. Once preheated, place casserole dish in the oven and close its lid.

NUTRITIONS: Calories 405   Total Fat 22.7 g   Saturated Fat 6.1 g   Cholesterol 4 mg   Sodium 227 mg   TotalCarbs26.1 g   Fiber 1.4 g Sugar 0.9 g   Protein 42 g

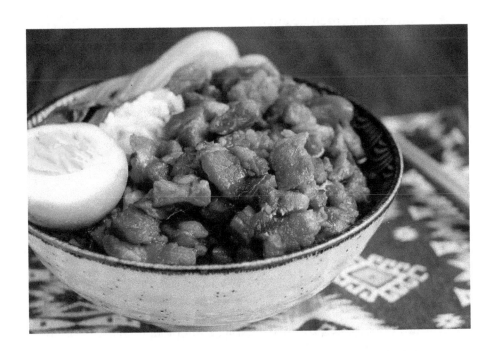

6. Pork Squash Bake

Preparation Time: 10 minutes

Cooking Time: 50 minutes

Serving: 6

INGREDIENTS

- ¼ cup olive oil
- 1 yellow squash, peeled and chopped
- 1 onion, diced
- 2 garlic cloves, crushed

- 1 lb. pork mince
- ½ teaspoon cinnamon
- ¼ teaspoon ground cumin
- 1 teaspoon fresh rosemary
- 2 cups tomato passata
- 2 oz. butter
- ¼ cup flour
- 2 cups almond milk
- ½ cup tasty cheese, grated
- 1 egg
- Salt and black pepper to taste

DIRECTIONS

1. Put a wok on moderate heat and add oil to heat.
2. Stir in squash, then sauté for 5 minutes.
3. Add pork, spices, rosemary, garlic, and onion, then stir cook for 8 minutes.
4. Stir in pasta, and tomato paste and cook on a simmer for 5 minutes.
5. Spread this pork mixture in a casserole dish.
6. Prepare the white sauce in a suitable pot.
7. Add oil to heat, then stir in flour and cook for 1 minute.
8. Pour in milk and stir cook until it thickens.
9. Stir in cheese, egg, salt, and black pepper.
10. Spread this white sauce over the pork pasta mixture.
11. Press "Power Button" of Air Fry Oven and turn the dial to select the "Bake" mode.
12. Press the Time button and again turn the dial to set the cooking time to 30 minutes.

13. Now push the Temp button and rotate the dial to set the temperature at 350 degrees F.
14. Once preheated, place casserole dish in the oven and close its lid.

NUTRITIONS:

Calories 545

Total Fat 36.4 g

Saturated Fat 10.1 g

Cholesterol 200 mg

Sodium 272 mg

Total Carbs 10.7 g

Fiber 0.2 g

Sugar 0.1 g

Protein 42.5 g

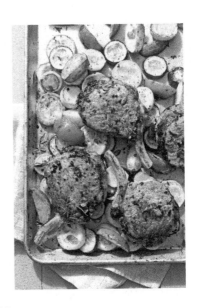

7. Cider Pork Skewers

Preparation Time: 10 minutes

Cooking Time: 15 minutes

Serving: 4

INGREDIENTS

- 3 garlic cloves, minced
- 4 tablespoon rapeseed oil
- 2 tablespoon cider vinegar
- Large bunch thyme
- 1 ¼ lb. boneless pork, diced

DIRECTIONS

1. Toss pork with all its thyme, oil, vinegar, and garlic.
2. Marinate the thyme pork for 2 hours in a closed container in the refrigerator.
3. Thread the marinated pork on the skewers.
4. Place these skewers in an Air fryer basket.
5. Press "Power Button" of Air Fry Oven and turn the dial to select the "Air fry" mode.
6. Press the Time button and again turn the dial to set the cooking time to 15 minutes.
7. Now push the Temp button and rotate the dial to set the temperature at 350 degrees F.
8. Once preheated, place the Air fryer basket in the oven and close its lid.
9. Flip the skewers when cooked halfway through then resume cooking.

10. Serve the skewers with salad.

NUTRITIONS: Calories 395 Total Fat 17.5 g Saturated Fat 4.8 g Cholesterol 283 mg Sodium 355 mg Total Carbs 26.4 g Fiber 1.8 g Sugar 0.8 g Protein 17.4 g

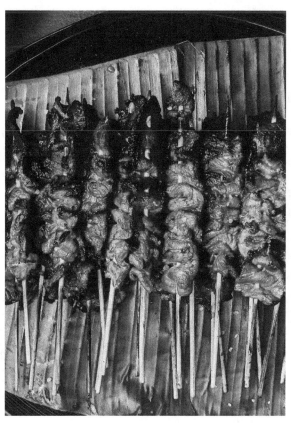

8.   <u>Mint Pork Kebobs</u>

Preparation Time: 10 minutes

Cooking Time: 15 minutes

Serving: 4

INGREDIENTS

- ½ cup cream
- 1½ tablespoon mint
- 1 teaspoon ground cumin
  - oz. diced pork
- ½ small onion, cubed
- 1 cup cottage cheese, cubed

DIRECTIONS

1. Whisk the cream with mint and cumin in a suitable bowl.
2. Toss in pork cubes and mix well to coat. Marinate for 30 minutes.
3. Alternatively, thread the pork, onion and cottage cheese on the skewers.
4. Place these pork skewers in the Air fry basket.
5. Press "Power Button" of Air Fry Oven and turn the dial to select the "Air fryer" mode.
6. Press the Time button and again turn the dial to set the cooking time to 15 minutes.
7. Now push the Temp button and rotate the dial to set the temperature at 370 degrees F.
8. Once preheated, place the Air fryer basket in the oven and close its lid.
9. Flip the skewers when cooked halfway through then resume cooking.

NUTRITIONS: Calories 311 Total Fat 8.9 g Saturated Fat 4.5 g Cholesterol 57 mg Sodium 340 mg Total Carbs24.7 g Fiber 1.2 g Sugar 1.3 g Protein 13 g

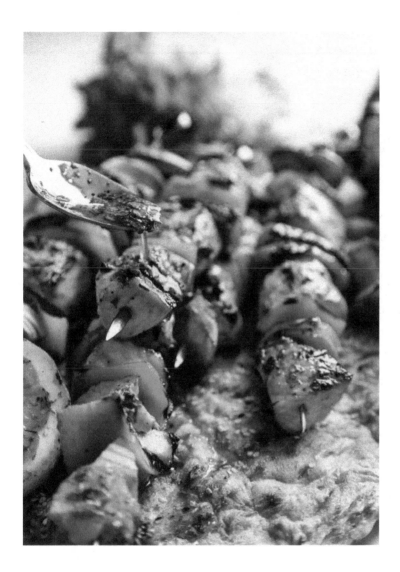

9.   <u>Tahini Pork Kebobs</u>

Preparation Time: 10 minutes

Cooking Time: 18 minutes

Serving: 6

INGREDIENTS

- 2 lbs. pork steaks
- 2 tablespoon tahini
- Zest and juice of 1 lemon
- 1 tablespoon maple syrup
- Handful thyme leaves, chopped

DIRECTIONS

1. Mix pork with tahini paste, lemon juice, zest, maple syrup and thyme.
2. Toss well to coat then marinate for 30 minutes.
3. Alternatively, thread the pork on the skewers.
4. Place these pork skewers in the Air fry basket.
5. Press "Power Button" of Air Fry Oven and turn the dial to select the "Air fryer" mode.
6. Press the Time button and again turn the dial to set the cooking time to 18 minutes.
7. Now push the Temp button and rotate the dial to set the temperature at 360 degrees F.
8. Once preheated, place the Air fryer basket in the oven and close its lid.
9. Flip the skewers when cooked halfway through then resume cooking.

NUTRITIONS: Calories 548 Total Fat 22.9 g Saturated Fat 9 g Cholesterol 105 mg Sodium 350 mg Total Carbs 17.5 g Sugar 10.9 g Fiber 6.3 g Protein 40.1 g

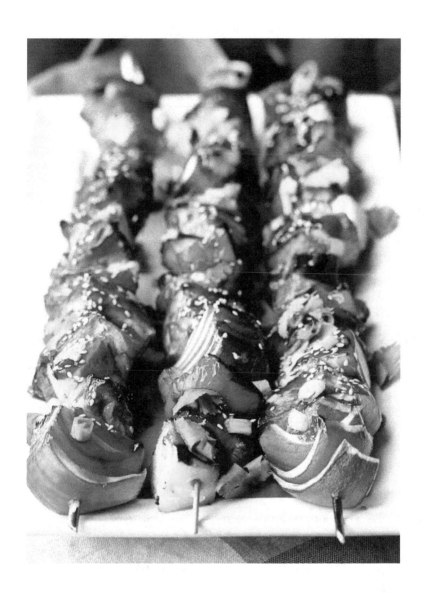

10. <u>Pork Skewers with Garden Salad</u>

Preparation Time: 10 minutes

Cooking Time: 20 minutes

Serving: 4

INGREDIENTS

- 1 ¼ lb. boneless pork, diced
- 2 teaspoons balsamic vinegar
- 2 tablespoons olive oil
- 1 garlic clove, crushed
- For the salad
- 4 large tomatoes, chopped
- 1 cucumber, chopped
- 1 handful black olives, chopped
- 9 oz. pack feta cheese, crumbled
- 1 bunch of parsley, chopped

DIRECTIONS

1. Whisk balsamic vinegar with garlic and olive oil in a bowl.
2. Toss in pork cubes and mix well to coat. Marinate for 30 minutes.
3. Alternatively, thread the pork on the skewers.
4. Place these pork skewers in the Air fry basket.
5. Press "Power Button" of Air Fry Oven and turn the dial to select the "Air fryer" mode.
6. Press the Time button and again turn the dial to set the cooking time to 20 minutes.
7. Now push the Temp button and rotate the dial to set the temperature at 360 degrees F.
8. Once preheated, place the Air fryer basket in the oven and close its lid.
9. Flip the skewers when cooked halfway through then resume cooking.
10. Meanwhile, whisk all the salad ingredients in a salad bowl.
11. Serve the skewers with prepared salad.

NUTRITIONS: Calories 289 Total Fat 50.5 g Saturated Fat 11.7 g Cholesterol 58 mg Sodium 463 mg Total Carbs 9.9 g Fiber 1.5 g Sugar 0.3 g Protein 29.3 g

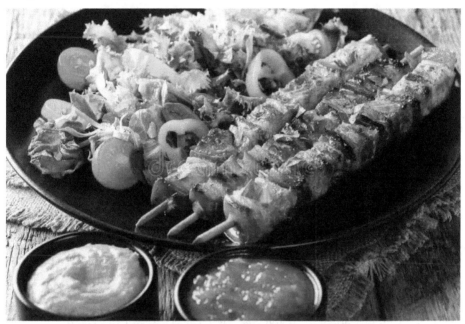

11. <u>Wine Soaked Pork Kebobs</u>

Preparation Time: 10 minutes

Cooking Time: 20 minutes

Serving: 6

INGREDIENTS

- 2 ¼ lbs. pork shoulder, diced
- 1/3 cup avocado oil
- ½ cup red wine

- 2 teaspoon dried oregano
- Zest and juice 2 limes
- 2 garlic cloves, crushed

DIRECTIONS

1. Whisk avocado oil, red wine, oregano, lime juice, zest, and garlic in a suitable bowl.
2. Toss in pork cubes and mix well to coat. Marinate for 30 minutes.
3. Alternatively, thread the pork, onion, and bread on the skewers.
4. Place these pork skewers in the Air fry basket.
5. Press "Power Button" of Air Fry Oven and turn the dial to select the "Air fryer" mode.
6. Press the Time button and again turn the dial to set the cooking time to 20 minutes.
7. Now push the Temp button and rotate the dial to set the temperature at 370 degrees F.
8. Once preheated, place the Air fryer basket in the oven and close its lid.
9. Flip the skewers when cooked halfway through then resume cooking.

NUTRITIONS: Calories 237 Total Fat 19.8 g Saturated Fat 1.4 g Cholesterol 10 mg Sodium 719 mg Total Carbs 1 g Fiber 0.9 g Sugar 1.4 g Protein 37.8

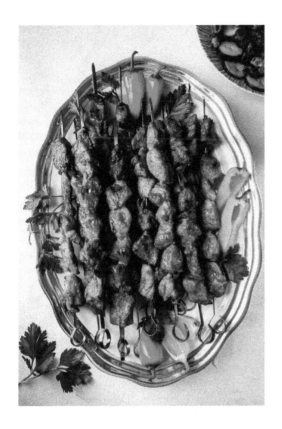

12. <u>Pork Sausages</u>

Preparation Time: 10 minutes

Cooking Time: 16 minutes

Serving: 6

INGREDIENTS

- 1 lb. pork mince
- 2 oz. feta cheese
- 1 large red onion, chopped
- ¼ cup parsley, chopped

- ¼ cup mint, chopped
- 1 tablespoon olive oil
- Juice 1 lemon

DIRECTIONS

1. Whisk pork mince with onion, feta, and everything in a bowl.
2. Make 12 sausages out of this mixture then thread them on the skewers.
3. Place these pork skewers in the Air fry basket.
4. Press "Power Button" of Air Fry Oven and turn the dial to select the "Bake" mode.
5. Press the Time button and again turn the dial to set the cooking time to 16 minutes.
6. Now push the Temp button and rotate the dial to set the temperature at 370 degrees F.
7. Once preheated, place the Air fryer basket in the oven and close its lid.
8. Flip the skewers when cooked halfway through then resume cooking.
9. Serve warm.

NUTRITIONS: Calories 452 Total Fat 4 g Saturated Fat 2 g Cholesterol 65 mg Sodium 220 mg Total Carbs23.1 g Fiber 0.3 g Sugar 1 g Protein 26g

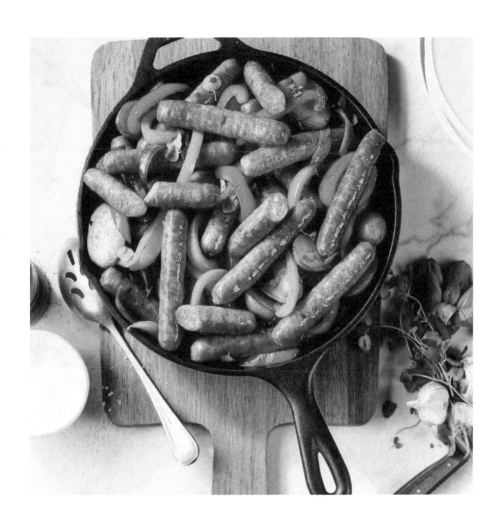

13. <u>Pest Pork Kebobs</u>

Preparation Time: 10 minutes

Cooking Time: 20 minutes

Serving: 4

INGREDIENTS

- 9 ½ oz. couscous, boiled

- 2 tablespoon pesto paste
- 2/3 lb. pork steak, diced
- 2 red peppers, cut into chunks
- 2 red onions, cut into chunks
- 1 tablespoon olive oil

DIRECTIONS

1. Toss in pork cubes with pesto and oil, then mix well to coat. Marinate for 30 minutes.
2. Alternatively, thread the pork, onion, and peppers on the skewers.
3. Place these pork skewers in the Air fry basket.
4. Press "Power Button" of Air Fry Oven and turn the dial to select the "Air fryer" mode.
5. Press the Time button and again turn the dial to set the cooking time to 20 minutes.
6. Now push the Temp button and rotate the dial to set the temperature at 370 degrees F.
7. Once preheated, place the Air fryer basket in the oven and close its lid.
8. Flip the skewers when cooked halfway through then resume cooking.
9. Serve warm with couscous.

NUTRITIONS: Calories 331 Total Fat 18 g Saturated Fat 2.7 g Cholesterol 75 mg Sodium 389 mg Total Carbs11.7 g Fiber 0.3g Sugar 0.1 g Protein 28.2 g

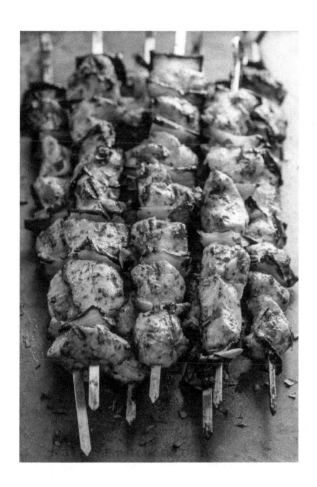

14. <u>**Pork Sausage with Yogurt Dip**</u>

Preparation Time: 10 minutes

Cooking Time: 10 minutes

Serving: 8

INGREDIENTS

- 2 tablespoon cumin seed
- 2 tablespoon coriander seed
- 2 tablespoon fennel seed

35

- 1 tablespoon paprika
- 4 garlic cloves, minced
- ½ teaspoon ground cinnamon
- 1 ½ lb. lean minced pork
- For the yogurt
- 3 zucchinis, grated
- 2 teaspoon cumin seed, toasted
- 9 0z. Greek yogurt
- Small handful chopped the coriander
- A small handful of chopped mint

DIRECTIONS

1. Blend all the spices and seeds with garlic and cinnamon in a blender.
2. Add this spice paste to the minced pork then mix well.
3. Make 8 sausages and thread each on the skewers.
4. Place these pork skewers in the Air fry basket.
5. Press "Power Button" of Air Fry Oven and turn the dial to select the "Air fryer" mode.
6. Press the Time button and again turn the dial to set the cooking time to 10 minutes.
7. Now push the Temp button and rotate the dial to set the temperature at 370 degrees F.
8. Once preheated, place the Air fryer basket in the oven and close its lid.
9. Flip the skewers when cooked halfway through then resume cooking.
10. Prepare the yogurt ingredients in a bowl.
11. Serve skewers with the yogurt mixture.

NUTRITIONS: Calories 341 Total Fat 20.5 g Saturated Fat 3 g Cholesterol 42 mg Sodium 688 mg Total Carbs 20.3 g Sugar 1.4 g Fiber 4.3 g Protein 49 g

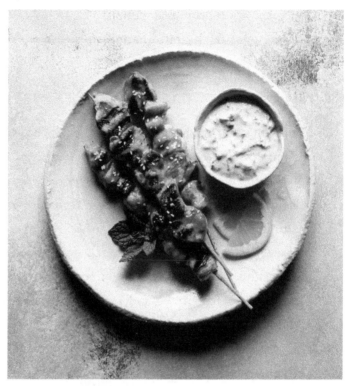

15. <u>Italian Parmesan Breaded Pork Chops</u>

Preparation Time: 5 minutes

Cooking Time: 25 minutes

Servings: 5

INGREDIENTS

- 5 (3½- to 5-ounce) pork chops (bone-in or boneless)
- 1 teaspoon Italian seasoning

- Seasoning salt
- Pepper
- ¼ cup all-purpose flour
- 2 tablespoons Italian bread crumbs
- 3 tablespoons finely grated Parmesan cheese
- Cooking oil

DIRECTIONS

1. Preparing the Ingredients. Season the pork chops with the Italian seasoning and seasoning salt and pepper to taste.
2. Sprinkle the flour on both sides of the pork chops, then coat both sides with the bread crumbs and Parmesan cheese.
3. Air Frying. Place the pork chops in the Air fryer oven. Stacking them is okay. Spray the pork chops with cooking oil. Set temperature to 360°F. Cook for 6 minutes.
4. Open the Air fryer oven and flip the pork chops. Cook for an additional 6 minutes.
5. Cool before serving. Instead of seasoning salt, you can use either chicken or pork rub for additional flavor. You can find these rubs in the spice aisle of the grocery store.

NUTRITIONS: Calories: 334Fat: 7GProtein: 34GFiber: 0G

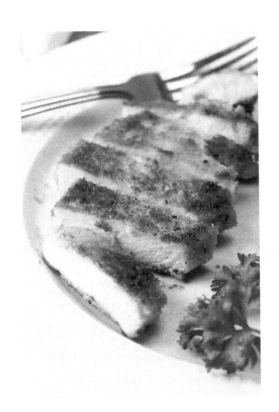

16. Crispy Breaded Pork Chops

Preparation Time: 10 minutes

Cooking Time: 15 minutes

Servings: 8

INGREDIENTS

- 1/8 tsp. pepper
- ¼ tsp. chili powder
- ½ tsp. onion powder
- ½ tsp. garlic powder

- 1 ¼ tsp. sweet paprika
- 2 tbsp. grated parmesan cheese
- 1/3 C. crushed cornflake crumbs
- ½ C. panko breadcrumbs
- 1 beaten egg
- 6 center-cut boneless pork chops

DIRECTIONS

1. Preparing the Ingredients. Ensure that your air fryer is preheated to 400 degrees. Spray the basket with olive oil.
2. With ½ teaspoon salt and pepper, season both sides of pork chops.
3. Combine ¾ teaspoon salt with pepper, chili powder, onion powder, garlic powder, paprika, cornflake crumbs, panko breadcrumbs, and parmesan cheese.
4. Beat egg in another bowl.
5. Dip pork chops into the egg and then crumb mixture.
6. Add pork chops to air fryer and spritz with olive oil.
7. Air Frying. Set temperature to 400°F, and set time to 12 minutes. Cook 12 minutes, making sure to flip over halfway through the cooking process.
8. Only add 3 chops in at a time and repeat the process with remaining pork chops.

NUTRITIONS: Calories: 378Fat: 13GProtein: 33GSugar: 1

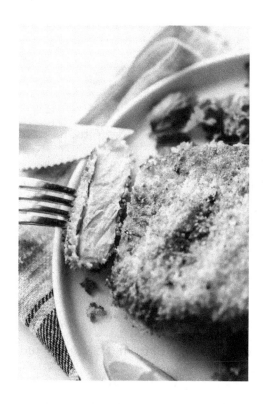

17. <u>Roasted Pork Tenderloin</u>

Preparation Time: 5 minutes

Cooking Time: 1 hour

Servings: 4

INGREDIENTS

- 1 (3-pound) pork tenderloin
- 2 tablespoons extra-virgin olive oil
- 2 garlic cloves, minced
- 1 teaspoon dried basil
- 1 teaspoon dried oregano
- 1 teaspoon dried thyme

- Salt
- Pepper

DIRECTIONS

1. Preparing the Ingredients. Drizzle the pork tenderloin with the olive oil.
2. Rub the garlic, basil, oregano, thyme, and salt and pepper to taste all over the tenderloin.
3. Air Frying. Place the tenderloin in the Air fryer oven. Cook for 45 minutes.
4. Use a meat thermometer to test for doneness
5. Open the Air fryer oven and flip the pork tenderloin. Cook for an additional 15 minutes.
6. Remove the cooked pork from the air fryer and allow it to rest for 10 minutes before cutting.

NUTRITIONS: Calories: 283Fat: 10GProtein: 48G

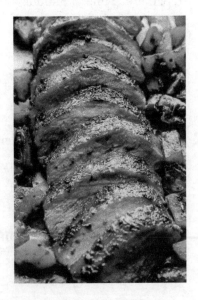

18. Bacon Wrapped Pork Tenderloin

Preparation Time: 5 minutes

Cooking Time: 15 minutes

Servings: 4

INGREDIENTS

- Pork:
- 1-2 tbsp. Dijon mustard
- 3-4 strips of bacon
- 1 pork tenderloin
- Apple Gravy:
- ½ - 1 tsp. Dijon mustard
- 1 tbsp. almond flour
- 2 tbsp. ghee
- 1 chopped onion
- 2-3 Granny Smith apples
- 1 C. vegetable broth

DIRECTIONS

1. Preparing the Ingredients. Spread Dijon mustard all over tenderloin and wrap the meat with strips of bacon.
2. Air Frying. Place into the Air fryer oven, set temperature to 360°F, and set time to 15 minutes and cook 10-15 minutes at 360 degrees. Use a meat thermometer to check for doneness.
3. To make sauce, heat ghee in a pan and add shallots. Cook 1-2 minutes.
4. Then add apples, cooking 3-5 minutes until softened.

5. Add flour and ghee to make a roux. Add broth and mustard, stirring well to combine.

6. When the sauce starts to bubble, add 1 cup of sautéed apples, cooking till sauce thickens.

7. Once pork tenderloin I cook, allow to sit 5-10 minutes to rest before slicing.

8. Serve topped with apple gravy.

NUTRITIONS: Calories: 552Fat: 25GProtein: 29G Sugar: 6G

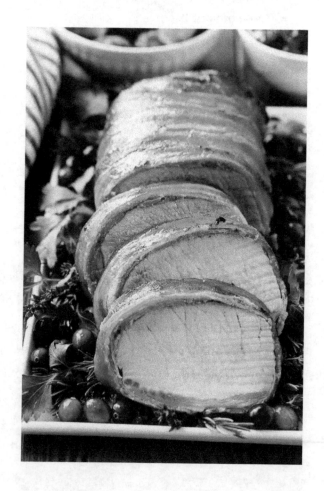

19. Dijon Garlic Pork Tenderloin

Preparation Time: 5 minutes

Cooking Time: 10 minutes

Servings: 6

INGREDIENTS

- 1 C. breadcrumbs
- Pinch of cayenne pepper
- 3 crushed garlic cloves
- 2 tbsp. ground ginger
- 2 tbsp. Dijon mustard
- 2 tbsp. raw honey
- 4 tbsp. water
- 2 tsp. salt
- 1 pound pork tenderloin, sliced into 1-inch rounds

DIRECTIONS

1. Preparing the Ingredients. With pepper and salt, season all sides of tenderloin.
2. Combine cayenne pepper, garlic, ginger, mustard, honey, and water until smooth.
3. Dip pork rounds into the honey mixture and then into breadcrumbs, ensuring they all get coated well.
4. Place coated pork rounds into your Air fryer oven.
5. Air Frying. Set temperature to 400°F, and set time to 10 minutes. Cook 10 minutes at 400 degrees. Flip and then cook an additional 5 minutes until golden in color.

NUTRITIONS: Calories: 423 Fat: 18G Protein: 31G Sugar: 3G

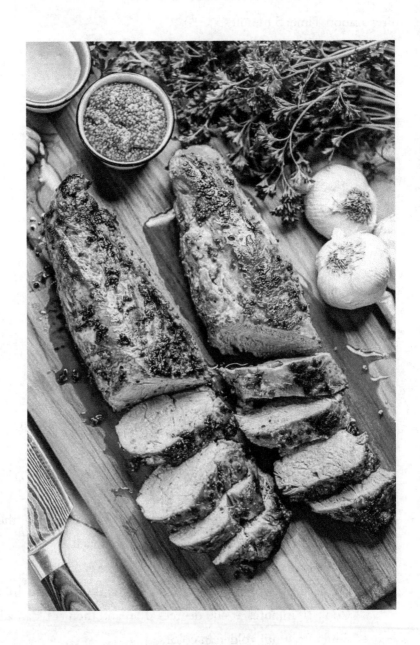

20. Air Fryer Sweet and Sour Pork

Preparation Time: 10 minutes

Cooking Time: 12 minutes

Servings: 6

INGREDIENTS

- 3 tbsp. olive oil
- 1/16 tsp. Chinese Five Spice
- ¼ tsp. pepper
- ½ tsp. sea salt
- 1 tsp. pure sesame oil
- 2 eggs
- 1 C. almond flour
- 2 pounds pork, sliced into chunks
- Sweet and Sour Sauce:
- ¼ tsp. sea salt
- ½ tsp. garlic powder
- 1 tbsp. low-sodium soy sauce
- ½ C. rice vinegar
- 5 tbsp. tomato paste
- 1/8 tsp. water
- ½ C. sweetener of choice

DIRECTIONS

1. Preparing the Ingredients. To make the dipping sauce, whisk all sauce ingredients together over medium heat, stirring 5 minutes. Simmer uncovered 5 minutes till thickened.
2. Meanwhile, combine almond flour, five spice, pepper, and salt.

3. In another bowl, mix eggs with sesame oil.
4. Dredge pork in flour mixture and then in egg mixture. Shake any excess off before adding to air fryer rack/basket.
5. Air Frying. Set temperature to 340°F, and set time to 12 minutes.
6. Serve with sweet and sour dipping sauce!

NUTRITIONS: Calories: 371 Fat: 17G Protein: 27G Sugar: 1G

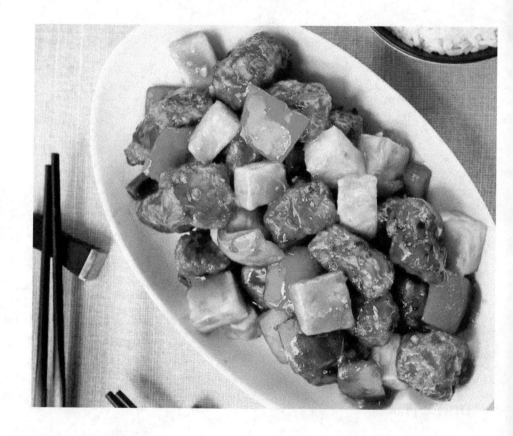

21. Teriyaki Pork Rolls

Preparation Time: 10 minutes

Cooking Time: 8 minutes

Servings: 6

INGREDIENTS

- 1 tsp. almond flour
- 4 tbsp. low-sodium soy sauce
- 4 tbsp. mirin
- 4 tbsp. brown sugar
- Thumb-sized amount of ginger, chopped
- Pork belly slices
- Enoki mushrooms

DIRECTIONS

1. Preparing the Ingredients. Mix brown sugar, mirin, soy sauce, almond flour, and ginger together until brown sugar dissolves.
2. Take pork belly slices and wrap around a bundle of mushrooms. Brush each roll with teriyaki sauce. Chill half an hour.
3. Preheat your Air fryer oven to 350 degrees and add marinated pork rolls.
4. Air Frying. Set temperature to 350°F, and set time to 8 minutes.

NUTRITIONS: Calories: 412 Fat: 9G Protein: 19G Sugar: 4G

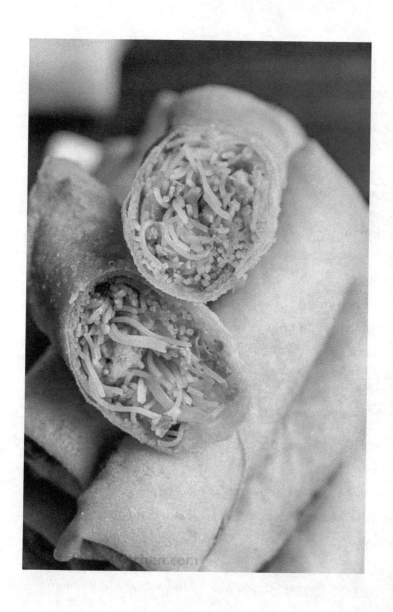

22. Rustic Pork Ribs

Preparation Time: 5 minutes

Cooking Time: 15 minutes

Servings: 4

INGREDIENTS

- 1 rack of pork ribs
- 3 tablespoons dry red wine
- 1 tablespoon soy sauce
- 1/2 teaspoon dried thyme
- 1/2 teaspoon onion powder
- 1/2 teaspoon garlic powder
- 1/2 teaspoon ground black pepper
- 1 teaspoon smoke salt
- 1 tablespoon cornstarch
- 1/2 teaspoon olive oil

DIRECTIONS

1. Preparing the Ingredients. Begin by preheating your Air fryer oven to 390 degrees F. Place all ingredients in a mixing bowl and let them marinate at least 1 hour.
2. Air Frying. Cook the marinated ribs approximately 25 minutes at 390 degrees F.
3. Serve hot.

NUTRITIONS: Calories: 249 Total Fat: 12.3g Sodium: 824mg Total Carbs: 3.2g Fiber: 0.2g Sugars: 0.4g Protein: 27.8g

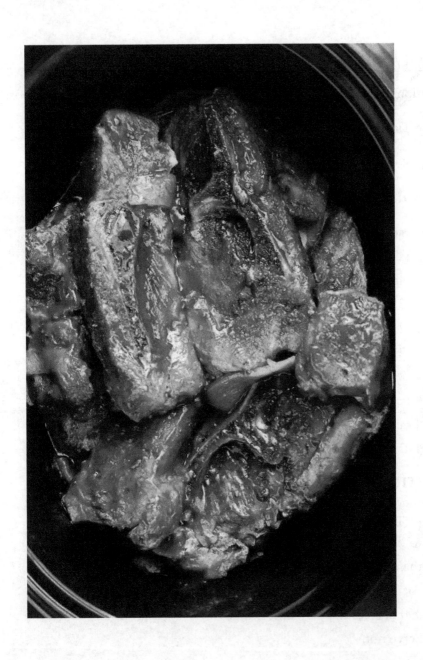

23. **Ginger, Garlic And Pork Dumplings**

Preparation Time: 10 minutes

Cooking Time: 15 minutes

Servings: 8

INGREDIENTS

- ¼ teaspoon crushed red pepper
- ½ teaspoon sugar
- 1 tablespoon chopped fresh ginger
- 1 tablespoon chopped garlic
- 1 teaspoon canola oil
- 1 teaspoon toasted sesame oil
- 18 dumpling wrappers
- 2 tablespoons rice vinegar
- 2 teaspoons soy sauce
- 4 cups bok choy, chopped
- 4 ounces ground pork

DIRECTIONS

1. Heat oil in a skillet and sauté the ginger and garlic until fragrant. Stir in the ground pork and cook for 5 minutes.
2. Stir in the bok choy and crushed red pepper. Season with salt and pepper to taste. Allow to cool.
3. Place the meat mixture in the middle of the dumpling wrappers. Fold the wrappers to seal the meat mixture in.
4. Place the bok choy in the grill pan.
5. Cook the dumplings in the air fryer at 330°F for 15 minutes.

6. Meanwhile, prepare the dipping sauce by combining the remaining Ingredients in a bowl.

NUTRITIONS: Calories: 137 Fat: 5G Protein: 7G

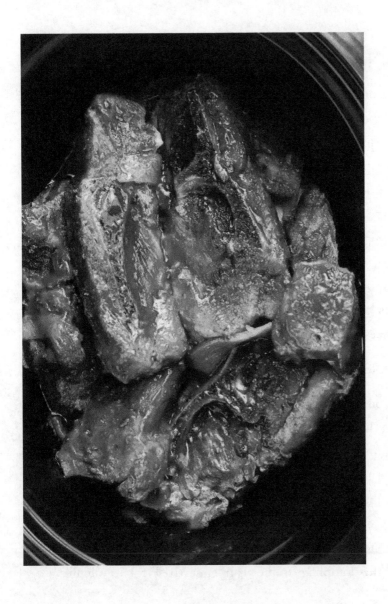

24. **Caramelized Pork Shoulder**

Preparation Time: 10 minutes

Cooking Time: 20 minutes

Servings: 8

INGREDIENTS

- 1/3 cup soy sauce
- 2 tablespoons sugar
- 1 tablespoon honey
- 2 pound pork shoulder, cut into 1½-inch thick slices

DIRECTIONS

1. In a bowl, mix together all ingredients except pork.
2. Add pork and coat with marinade generously.
3. Cover and refrigerate o marinate for about 2-8 hours.
4. Preheat the Cosori Air Fryer Oven to 335 degrees F.
5. Place the pork in an Air fryer basket.
6. Cook for about 10 minutes.
7. Now, set the Cosori Air Fryer Oven to 390 degrees F. Cook for about 10 minutes

NUTRITIONS: Calories: 356 Total Fat: 24.3g Sodium: 676mg Total Carbs: 6g Fiber: 0.1g Sugars: 5.3g Protein: 27.1g

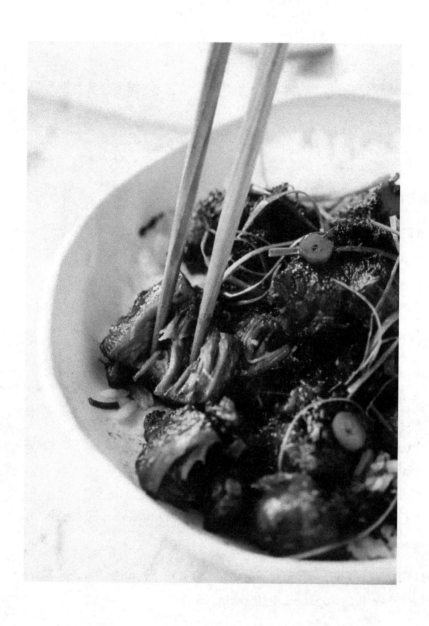

25. **Curry Pork Roast in Coconut Sauce**

Preparation Time: 10 minutes

Cooking Time: 60 minutes

Servings: 6

INGREDIENTS

- ½ teaspoon curry powder
- ½ teaspoon ground turmeric powder
- 1 can unsweetened coconut milk
- 1 tablespoons sugar
- 2 tablespoons fish sauce
- 2 tablespoons soy sauce
- 3 pounds pork shoulder
- Salt and pepper to taste

DIRECTIONS

1. Place all Ingredients in bowl and allow the meat to marinate in the fridge for at least 2 hours.
2. Preheat the air fryer to 390°F.
3. Place the grill pan accessory in the air fryer.
4. Grill the meat for 20 minutes making sure to flip the pork every 10 minutes for even grilling and cook in batches.
5. Meanwhile, pour the marinade in a saucepan and allow to simmer for 10 minutes until the sauce thickens.
6. Baste the pork with the sauce before serving.

NUTRITIONS: Calories: 688 Fat: 52G Protein: 17G

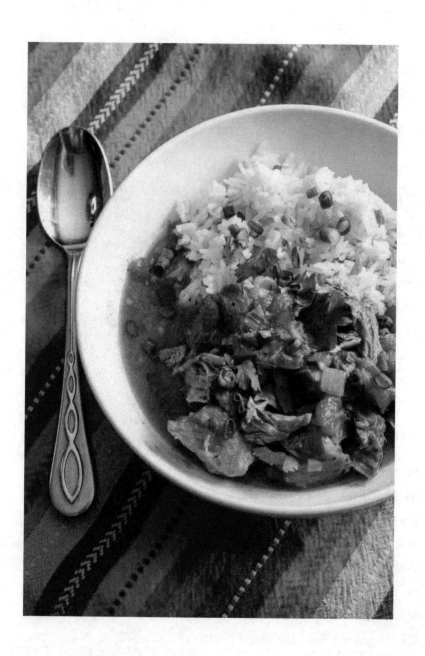

26.   Chinese Salt and Pepper Pork Chop Stir-fry

Preparation Time: 10 minutes

Cooking Time: 15 minutes

Servings: 4

INGREDIENTS

- Pork Chops:
- Olive oil
- ¾ C. almond flour
- ¼ tsp. pepper
- ½ tsp. salt
- 1 egg white
- Pork Chops
- Stir-fry:
- ¼ tsp. pepper
- 1 tsp. sea salt
- 2 tbsp. olive oil
- 2 sliced scallions
- 2 sliced jalapeno peppers

DIRECTIONS

1. Coat the Cosori Air Fryer Oven basket with olive oil.
2. Whisk pepper, salt, and egg white together till foamy.
3. Cut pork chops into pieces, leaving just a bit on bones. Pat dry.
4. Add pieces of pork to egg white mixture, coating well. Let sit for marinade 20 minutes.
5. Put marinated chops into a large bowl and add almond flour. Dredge and shake off excess and place into air fryer.

6. Set temperature to 360°F, and set time to 12 minutes. Cook 12 minutes at 360 degrees.

7. Turn up the heat to 400 degrees and cook another 6 minutes till pork chops are nice and crisp.

8. To make stir-fry, remove jalapeno seeds and chop up. Chop scallions and mix with jalapeno pieces.

9. Heat a skillet with olive oil. Stir-fry pepper, salt, scallions, and jalapenos 60 seconds. Then add fried pork pieces to skills and toss with scallion mixture. Stir-fry 1-2 minutes till well coated and hot.

NUTRITIONS: Calories: 294 Fat: 17G Protein: 36G Sugar: 4G

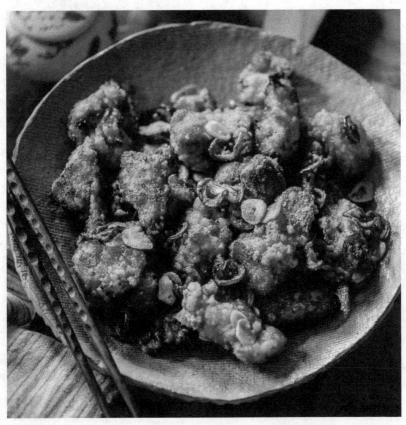

27. **Roasted Pork Tenderloin**

Preparation Time: 5 minutes

Cooking Time: 1 hour

Servings: 4

INGREDIENTS

- 1 (3-pound) pork tenderloin
- 2 tablespoons extra-virgin olive oil
- 2 garlic cloves, minced
- 1 teaspoon dried basil
- 1 teaspoon dried oregano
- 1 teaspoon dried thyme
- Salt
- Pepper

DIRECTIONS

1. Drizzle the pork tenderloin with the olive oil.
2. Rub the garlic, basil, oregano, thyme, and salt and pepper to taste all over the tenderloin.
3. Pour into the Oven rack/basket. Place the Rack on the middle-shelf of the Cosori Air Fryer Oven. Set temperature to 350°F, and set time to 45 minutes. Use a meat thermometer to test for doneness
4. Open the air fryer and flip the pork tenderloin. Cook for an additional 15 minutes.
5. Remove the cooked pork from the air fryer and allow it to rest for 10 minutes before cutting.

NUTRITIONS: Calories: 283 Fat: 10G Protein: 48G

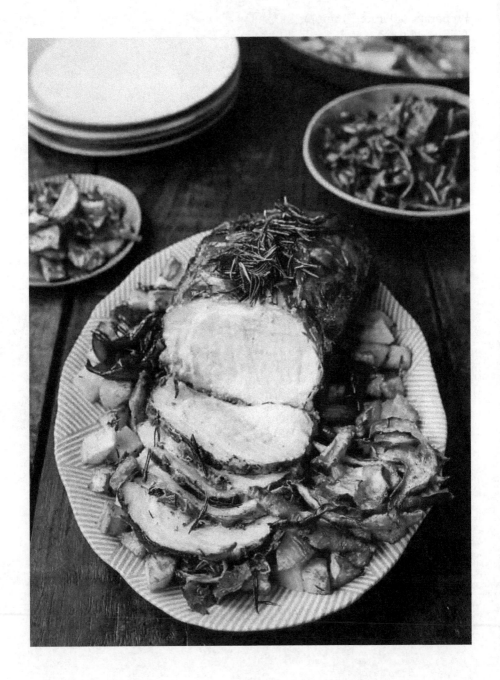

28. **Garlic Putter Pork Chops**

Preparation Time: 10 minutes

Cooking Time: 7 minutes

Servings: 4

INGREDIENTS

- 2 tsp. parsley
- 2 tsp. grated garlic cloves
- 1 tbsp. coconut oil
- 1 tbsp. coconut butter
- 4 pork chops

DIRECTIONS

1. Ensure your Cosori Air Fryer Oven is preheated to 350 degrees.
2. Mix butter, coconut oil, and all seasoning together. Then rub seasoning mixture over all sides of pork chops. Place in foil, seal, and chill for 1 hour.
3. Remove pork chops from foil and place into air fryer.
4. Pour into the Oven rack/basket. Place the Rack on the middle-shelf of the Cosori Air Fryer Oven. Set temperature to 350°F, and set time to 7 minutes. Cook 7 minutes on one side and 8 minutes on the other.
5. Drizzle with olive oil and serve alongside a green salad.

NUTRITIONS: Calories: 526 Fat: 23G Protein: 41G Sugar: 4G

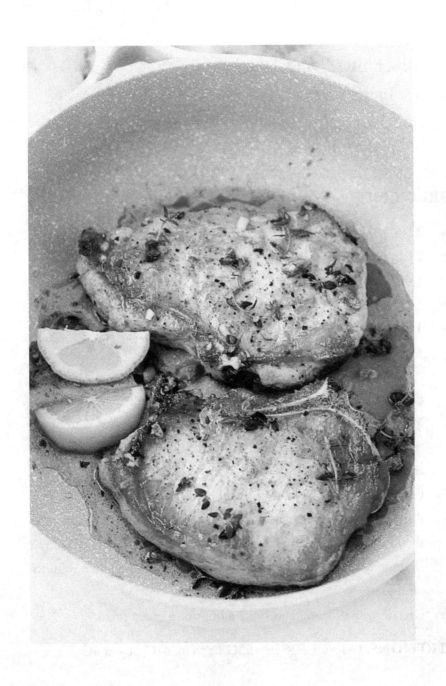

29. **Fried Pork with Sweet and Sour Glaze**

Preparation Time: 5 minutes

Cooking Time: 30 minutes

Servings: 4

INGREDIENTS

- ¼ cup rice wine vinegar
- ¼ teaspoon Chinese five spice powder
- 1 cup potato starch
- 1 green onion, chopped
- 2 large eggs, beaten
- 2 pounds pork chops cut into chunks
- 2 tablespoons cornstarch + 3 tablespoons water
- 5 tablespoons brown sugar
- Salt and pepper to taste

DIRECTIONS

1. Preheat the Cosori Air Fryer Oven to 390°F.
2. Season pork chops with salt and pepper to taste.
3. Dip the pork chops in egg. Set aside.
4. In a bowl, combine the potato starch and Chinese five spice powder.
5. Dredge the pork chops in the flour mixture.
6. Place in the double layer rack and cook for 30 minutes.
7. Meanwhile, place the vinegar and brown sugar in a saucepan. Season with salt and pepper to taste. Stir in the cornstarch slurry and allow to simmer until thick.
8. Serve the pork chops with the sauce and garnish with green onions.

NUTRITIONS: Calories: 420 Fat: 11.8G Protein: 69.2G

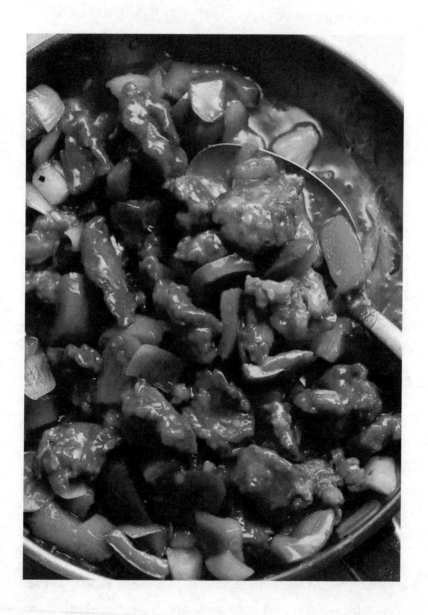

30. Oregano-Paprika on Breaded Pork

Preparation Time: 10 minutes

Cooking Time: 30 minutes

Servings: 4

INGREDIENTS

- ¼ cup water
- ¼ teaspoon dry mustard
- ½ teaspoon black pepper
- ½ teaspoon cayenne pepper
- ½ teaspoon garlic powder
- ½ teaspoon salt
- 1 cup panko breadcrumbs
- 1 egg, beaten
- 2 teaspoons oregano
- 4 lean pork chops
- 4 teaspoons paprika

DIRECTIONS

1. Preheat the Cosori Air Fryer Oven to 390°F.
2. Pat dry the pork chops.
3. In a mixing bowl, combine the egg and water. Then set aside.
4. In another bowl, combine the rest of the Ingredients.
5. Dip the pork chops in the egg mixture and dredge in the flour mixture.
6. Place in the air fryer basket and cook for 25 to 30 minutes until golden.

NUTRITIONS: Calories: 364Fat: 20.2GProtein: 42.9G

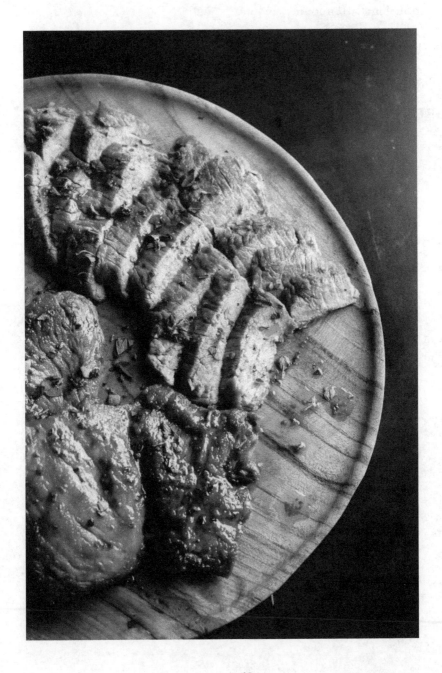

31. **Bacon Wrapped Pork Tenderloin**

Preparation Time: 5 minutes

Cooking Time: 15 minutes

Servings: 4

INGREDIENTS

- Pork:
- 1-2 tbsp. Dijon mustard
- 3-4 strips of bacon
- 1 pork tenderloin
- Apple Gravy:
- ½ - 1 tsp. Dijon mustard
- 1 tbsp. almond flour
- 2 tbsp. ghee
- 1 chopped onion
- 2-3 Granny Smith apples
- 1 C. vegetable broth

DIRECTIONS

1. Spread Dijon mustard all over tenderloin and wrap meat with strips of bacon.
2. Pour into the Oven rack/basket. Place the Rack on the middle-shelf of the Cosori Air Fryer Oven. Set temperature to 360°F, and set time to 15 minutes. Use a meat thermometer to check for doneness.
3. To make sauce, heat ghee in a pan and add shallots. Cook 1-2 minutes.
4. Then add apples, cooking 3-5 minutes until softened.

5. Add flour and ghee to make a roux. Add broth and mustard, stirring well to combine.

6. When sauce starts to bubble, add 1 cup of sautéed apples, cooking till sauce thickens.

7. Once pork tenderloin I cook, allow to sit 5-10 minutes to rest before slicing.

8. Serve topped with apple gravy. Devour!

NUTRITIONS: Calories: 552Fat: 25G Protein: 29G Sugar: 6G

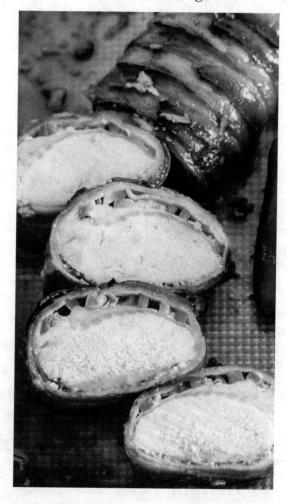

32. **Dijon Garlic Pork Tenderloin**

Preparation Time: 5 minutes

Cooking Time: 10 minutes

Servings: 6

INGREDIENTS

- 1 C. breadcrumbs
- Pinch of cayenne pepper
- 3 crushed garlic cloves
- 2 tbsp. ground ginger
- 2 tbsp. Dijon mustard
- 2 tbsp. raw honey
- 4 tbsp. water
- 2 tsp. salt
- 1 pound pork tenderloin, sliced into 1-inch rounds

DIRECTIONS

1. With pepper and salt, season all sides of tenderloin.
2. Combine cayenne pepper, garlic, ginger, mustard, honey, and water until smooth.
3. Dip pork rounds into honey mixture and then into breadcrumbs, ensuring they all get coated well.
4. Place coated pork rounds into your Cosori Air Fryer Oven.
5. Pour into the Oven rack/basket. Place the Rack on the middle-shelf of the Cosori Air Fryer Oven. Set temperature to 400°F, and set time to 10 minutes. Cook 10 minutes at 400 degrees. Flip and then cook an additional 5 minutes until golden in color.

NUTRITIONS: Calories: 423 Fat: 18G Protein: 31G Sugar: 3G

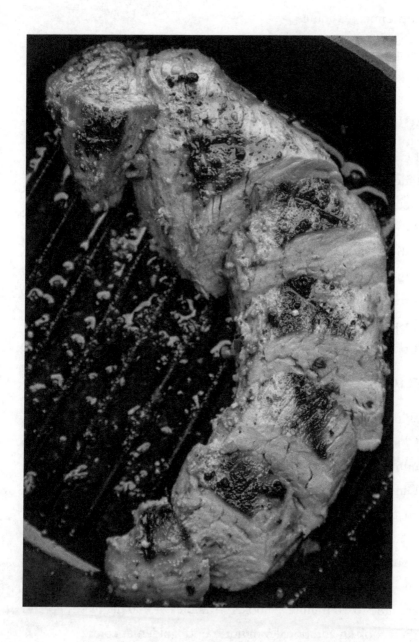

33. **Pork Neck with Salad**

Preparation Time: 10 minutes

Cooking Time: 12 minutes

Servings: 2

INGREDIENTS

- For Pork:
- 1 tablespoon soy sauce
- 1 tablespoon fish sauce
- ½ tablespoon oyster sauce
- ½ pound pork neck
- For Salad:
- 1 ripe tomato, sliced tickly
- 8-10 Thai shallots, sliced
- 1 scallion, chopped
- 1 bunch fresh basil leaves
- 1 bunch fresh cilantro leaves
- For Dressing:
- 3 tablespoons fish sauce
- 2 tablespoons olive oil
- 1 teaspoon apple cider vinegar
- 1 tablespoon palm sugar
- 2 bird eye chili
- 1 tablespoon garlic, minced

DIRECTIONS

1. For pork in a bowl, mix together all ingredients except pork.

2. Add pork neck and coat with marinade evenly. Refrigerate for about 2-3 hours.
3. Preheat the Cosori Air Fryer Oven to 340 degrees F.
4. Place the pork neck onto a grill pan. Cook for about 12 minutes.
5. Meanwhile in a large salad bowl, mix together all salad ingredients.
6. In a bowl, add all dressing ingredients and beat till well combined.
7. Remove pork neck from Air fryer and cut into desired slices.
8. Place pork slices over salad.

NUTRITIONS: Calories: 214 Total Fat: 17.1g Sodium: 1181mg Total Carbs: 11.2g Fiber: 0.7g   Sugars: 1.5g Protein: 6.4g

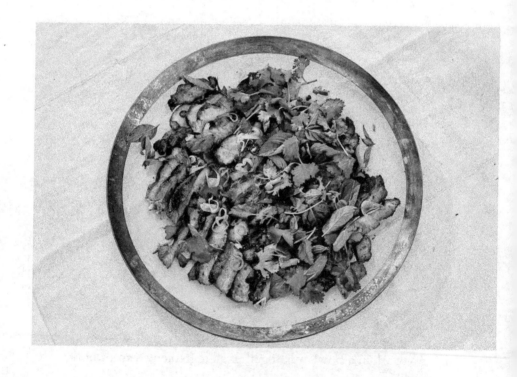

34. **Cajun Pork Steaks**

Preparation Time: 5 minutes

Cooking Time: 20 minutes

Servings: 6

INGREDIENTS

- 4-6 pork steaks
- BBQ sauce:
- Cajun seasoning
- 1 tbsp. vinegar
- 1 tsp. low-sodium soy sauce
- ½ C. brown sugar
- ½ C. vegan ketchup

DIRECTIONS

1. Ensure your Cosori Air Fryer Oven is preheated to 290 degrees.
2. Sprinkle pork steaks with Cajun seasoning.
3. Combine remaining ingredients and brush onto steaks. Add coated steaks to air fryer.
4. Pour into the Oven rack/basket. Place the Rack on the middle-shelf of the Cosori Air Fryer Oven. Set temperature to 290°F, and set time to 20 minutes. Cook 15-20 minutes till just browned.

NUTRITIONS: Calories: 209 Fat: 11G Protein: 28G Sugar: 2G

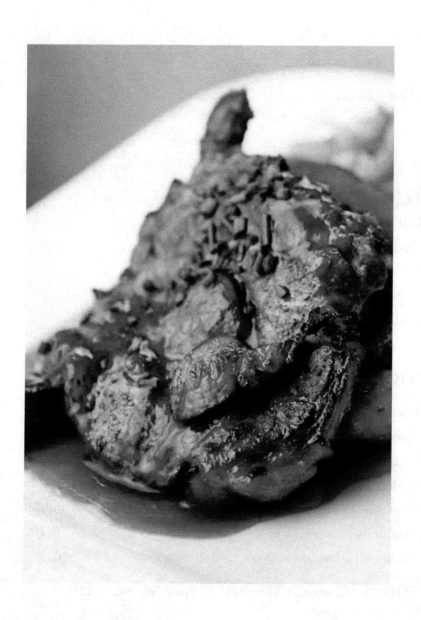

35. Cajun Sweet-Sour Grilled Pork

Preparation Time: 5 minutes

Cooking Time: 12 minutes

Servings: 3

INGREDIENTS

- ¼ cup brown sugar
- 1/4 cup cider vinegar
- 1-lb pork loin, sliced into 1-inch cubes
- 2 tablespoons Cajun seasoning
- 3 tablespoons brown sugar

DIRECTIONS

1. In a shallow dish, mix well pork loin, 3 tablespoons brown sugar, and Cajun seasoning. Toss well to coat. Marinate in the ref for 3 hours.
2. In a medium bowl mix well, brown sugar and vinegar for basting.
3. Thread pork pieces in skewers. Baste with sauce and place on skewer rack in air fryer.
4. For 12 minutes, cook on 360°F. Halfway through cooking time, turnover skewers and baste with sauce. If needed, cook in batches.
5. Serve and enjoy.

NUTRITIONS: Calories: *428* Fat: 16.7G Protein: 39G Sugar: 2G

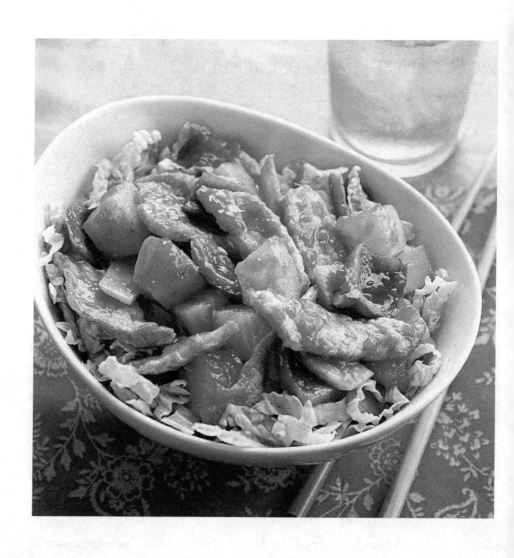

36. **Chinese Braised Pork Belly**

Preparation Time: 5 minutes

Cooking Time: 20 minutes

Servings: 8

INGREDIENTS

- 1 lb Pork Belly, sliced
- 1 Tbsp Oyster Sauce
- 1 Tbsp Sugar
- 2 Red Fermented Bean Curds
- 1 Tbsp Red Fermented Bean Curd Paste
- 1 Tbsp Cooking Wine
- 1/2 Tbsp Soy Sauce
- 1 Tsp Sesame Oil
- 1 Cup All Purpose Flour

DIRECTIONS

1. Preheat the Cosori Air Fryer Oven to 390 degrees.
2. In a small bowl, mix all ingredients together and rub the pork thoroughly with this mixture
3. Set aside to marinate for at least 30 minutes or preferably overnight for the flavors to permeate the meat
4. Coat each marinated pork belly slice in flour and place in the air fryer tray
5. Cook for 15 to 20 minutes until crispy and tender.

NUTRITIONS: Calories: 332 Total Fat: 16g Sodium: 986mg Total Carbs: 13.6g Fiber: 0.4g   Sugars: 1.6g Protein: 27.9g

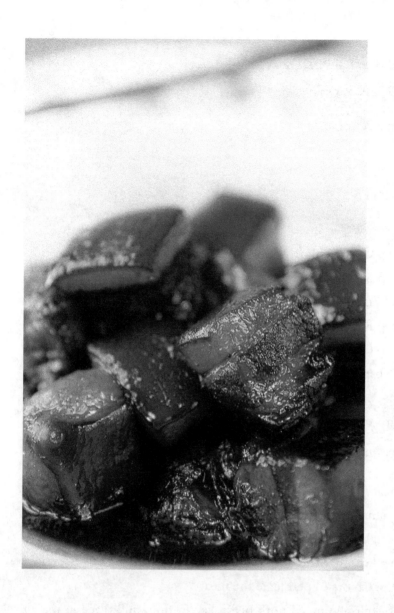

37. **Air Fryer Sweet and Sour Pork**

Preparation Time: 10 minutes

Cooking Time: 12 minutes

Servings: 6

INGREDIENTS

- 3 tbsp. olive oil
- 1/16 tsp. Chinese Five Spice
- ¼ tsp. pepper
- ½ tsp. sea salt
- 1 tsp. pure sesame oil
- 2 eggs
- 1 C. almond flour
- 2 pounds pork, sliced into chunks
- Sweet and Sour Sauce:
- ¼ tsp. sea salt
- ½ tsp. garlic powder
- 1 tbsp. low-sodium soy sauce
- ½ C. rice vinegar
- 5 tbsp. tomato paste
- 1/8 tsp. water
- ½ C. sweetener of choice

DIRECTIONS

1. To make the dipping sauce, whisk all sauce ingredients together over medium heat, stirring 5 minutes. Simmer uncovered 5 minutes till thickened.
2. Meanwhile, combine almond flour, five spice, pepper, and salt.

3. In another bowl, mix eggs with sesame oil.

4. Dredge pork in flour mixture and then in egg mixture. Shake any excess off before adding to air fryer basket.

5. Pour into the Oven rack/basket. Place the Rack on the middle-shelf of the Cosori Air Fryer Oven. Set temperature to 340°F, and set time to 12 minutes. Serve with sweet and sour dipping sauce.

NUTRITIONS: Calories: 371 Fat: 17G Protein: 27G Sugar: 1G

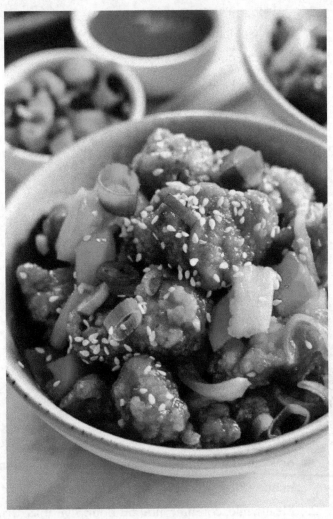

38. **Pork Loin with Potatoes**

Preparation Time: 10 minutes

Cooking Time: 25 minutes

Servings: 2

INGREDIENTS

- 2 pounds pork loin
- 1 teaspoon fresh parsley, chopped
- 2 large red potatoes, chopped
- ½ teaspoon garlic powder
- ½ teaspoon red pepper flakes, crushed
- Salt and freshly ground black pepper, to taste

DIRECTIONS

1. In a large bowl, add all ingredients except glaze and toss to coat well. Preheat the Cosori Air Fryer Oven to 325 degrees F. Place the loin in the air fryer basket.
2. Arrange the potatoes around pork loin.
3. Cook for about 25 minutes.

NUTRITIONS: Calories: 1360 Total Fat: 63.8g Sodium: 304mg Total Carbs: 59.5g Fiber: 6.5g   Sugars: 3.9g Protein: 131.1g

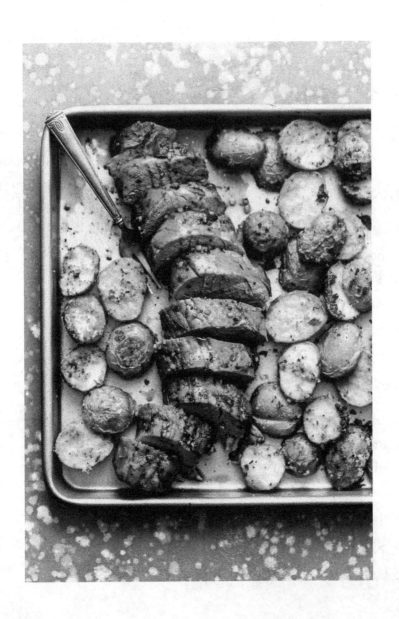

39. **Fried Pork Scotch Egg**

Preparation Time: 10 minutes

Cooking Time: 25 minutes

Servings: 2

INGREDIENTS

- 3 soft-boiled eggs, peeled
- 8 ounces of raw minced pork, or sausage outside the casings
- 2 teaspoons of ground rosemary
- 2 teaspoons of garlic powder
- Pinch of salt and pepper
- 2 raw eggs
- 1 cup of breadcrumbs (Panko, but other brands are fine, or home-made bread crumbs work too)

DIRECTIONS

1. Cover the basket of the air fryer with a lining of tin foil, leaving the edges uncovered to allow air to circulate through the basket. Preheat the Cosori Air Fryer Oven to 350 degrees.
2. In a mixing bowl, combine the raw pork with the rosemary, garlic powder, salt and pepper. This will probably be easiest to do with your masher or bare hands (though make sure to wash thoroughly after handling raw meat!); combine until all the spices are evenly spread throughout the meat.
3. Divide the meat mixture into three equal portions in the mixing bowl, and form each into balls with your hands.
4. Lay a large sheet of plastic wrap on the countertop, and flatten one of the balls of meat on top of it, to form a wide, flat meat-circle.

5. Place one of the peeled soft-boiled eggs in the center of the meat-circle and then, using the ends of the plastic wrap, pull the meat-circle so that it is fully covering and surrounding the soft-boiled egg.

6. Tighten and shape the plastic wrap covering the meat so that if forms a ball, and make sure not to squeeze too hard lest you squish the soft-boiled egg at the center of the ball! Set aside.

7. Repeat steps 5-7 with the other two soft-boiled eggs and portions of meat-mixture.

8. In a separate mixing bowl, beat the two raw eggs until fluffy and until the yolks and whites are fully combined.

9. One by one, remove the plastic wrap and dunk the pork-covered balls into the raw egg, and then roll them in the bread crumbs, covering fully and generously.

10. Place each of the bread-crumb covered meat-wrapped balls onto the foil-lined surface of the air fryer. Three of them should fit nicely, without touching.

11. Set the Cosori Air Fryer Oven timer to 25 minutes.

12. About halfway through the cooking time, shake the handle of the air-fryer vigorously, so that the scotch eggs inside roll around and ensure full coverage.

13. After 25 minutes, the air fryer will shut off and the scotch eggs should be perfect – the meat fully cooked, the egg-yolks still runny on the inside, and the outsides crispy and golden-brown. Using tongs, place them on serving plates, slice in half, and enjoy

NUTRITIONS: Calories: 578 Total Fat: 25g Sodium: 541mg Total Carbs: 43.6g Fiber: 3.2g   Sugars: 5.9g Protein: 43.6g

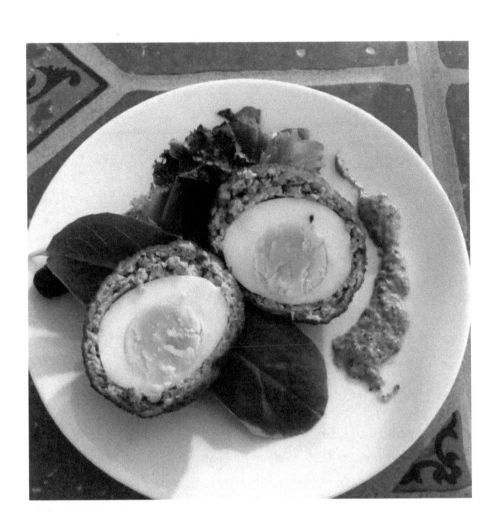

40. **Roasted Char Siew (Pork Butt)**

Preparation Time: 10 minutes

Cooking Time: 25 minutes

Servings: 6

INGREDIENTS

- 1 strip of pork shoulder butt with a good amount of fat marbling
- Marinade:
- 1 tsp. sesame oil
- 4 tbsp. raw honey
- 1 tsp. low-sodium dark soy sauce
- 1 tsp. light soy sauce
- 1 tbsp. rose wine
- 2 tbsp. Hoisin sauce

DIRECTIONS

1. Combine all marinade ingredients together and add to Ziploc bag. Place pork in bag, making sure all sections of pork strip are engulfed in the marinade. Chill 3-24 hours.
2. Take out the strip 30 minutes before planning to cook and preheat your Cosori Air Fryer Oven to 350 degrees.
3. Place foil on small pan and brush with olive oil. Place marinated pork strip onto prepared pan.
4. Set temperature to 350°F, and set time to 20 minutes. Roast 20 minutes.
5. Glaze with marinade every 5-10 minutes.
6. Remove strip and leave to cool a few minutes before slicing.

NUTRITIONS: Calories: 289 Fat: 13G Protein: 33G Sugar: 1G

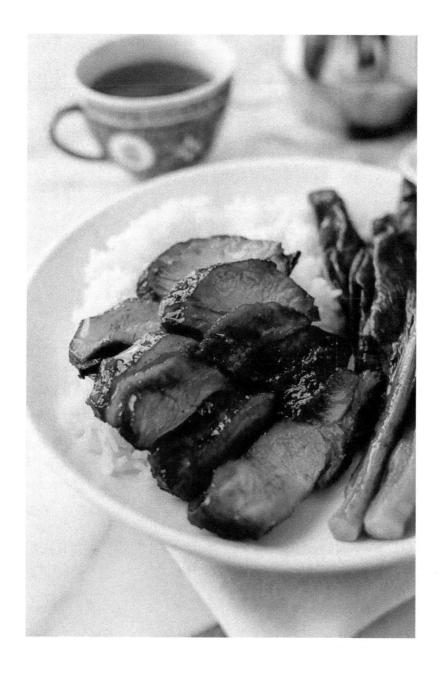

41. **Juicy Pork Ribs Ole**

Preparation Time: 10 minutes

Cooking Time: 25 minutes

Servings: 4

INGREDIENTS

- 1 rack of pork ribs
- 1/2 cup low-fat milk
- 1 tablespoon envelope taco seasoning mix
- 1 can tomato sauce
- 1/2 teaspoon ground black pepper
- 1 teaspoon seasoned salt
- 1 tablespoon cornstarch
- 1 teaspoon canola oil

DIRECTIONS

1. Place all ingredients in a mixing dish; let them marinate for 1 hour.
2. Pour into the Oven rack/basket. Place the Rack on the middle-shelf of the Cosori Air Fryer Oven. Set temperature to 390°F, and set time to 25 minutes. Cook the marinated ribs approximately 25 minutes.
3. Work with batches. Enjoy

NUTRITIONS: Calories: 181 Total Fat: 11.2g Sodium: 611mg Total Carbs: 3.4g Fiber: 0g   Sugars: 1.6g Protein: 16g

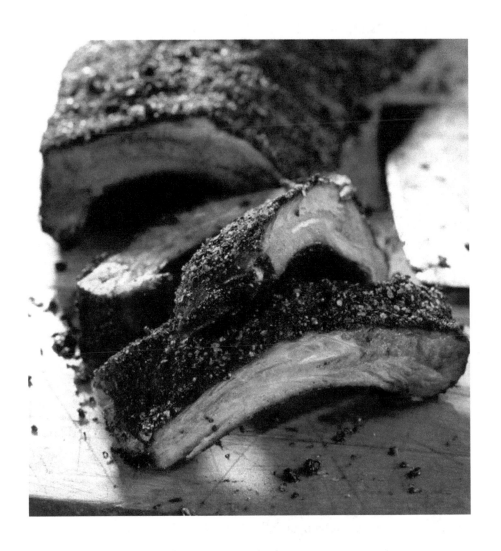

42. **Asian Pork Chops**

Preparation Time: 2 hours and 10 minutes

Cooking Time: 15 minutes

Servings: 4

INGREDIENTS

- 1/2 cup hoisin sauce
- 3 tablespoons cider vinegar
- 1 tablespoon Asian sweet chili sauce
- 1/4 teaspoon garlic powder
- 4 (1/2-inch-thick) boneless pork chops
- 1 teaspoon salt
- 1/2 teaspoon pepper

DIRECTIONS

1. Stir together hoisin, chili sauce, garlic powder, and vinegar in a large mixing bowl. Separate 1/4 cup of this mixture, then add pork chops to the bowl and marinate in the fridge for 2 hours. Remove the pork chops and place them on a plate. Sprinkle each side of the pork chop evenly with salt and pepper.
2. Pour into the Oven rack/basket. Place the Rack on the middle-shelf of the Cosori Air Fryer Oven. Set temperature to 360°F, and set time to 14 minutes. Cook for 14 minutes, flipping half way through. Brush with reserved marinade and serve.

NUTRITIONS: Calories: 338 Fat: 21G Protein: 19G Fiber: 1G

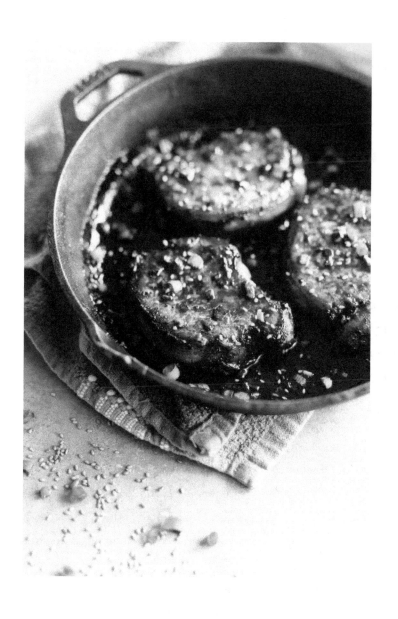

43. **Teriyaki Pork Rolls**

Preparation Time: 10 minutes

Cooking Time: 8 minutes

Servings: 6

INGREDIENTS

- 1 tsp. almond flour
- 4 tbsp. low-sodium soy sauce
- 4 tbsp. mirin
- 4 tbsp. brown sugar
- Thumb-sized amount of ginger, chopped
- Pork belly slices
- Enoki mushrooms

DIRECTIONS

1. Mix brown sugar, mirin, soy sauce, almond flour, and ginger together until brown sugar dissolves.
2. Take pork belly slices and wrap around a bundle of mushrooms. Brush each roll with teriyaki sauce. Chill half an hour.
3. Preheat your Cosori Air Fryer Oven to 350 degrees and add marinated pork rolls.
4. Pour into the Oven rack/basket. Place the Rack on the middle-shelf of the Cosori Air Fryer Oven. Set temperature to 350°F, and set time to 8 minutes.

NUTRITIONS: Calories: 412 Fat: 9G Protein: 19G Sugar: 4G

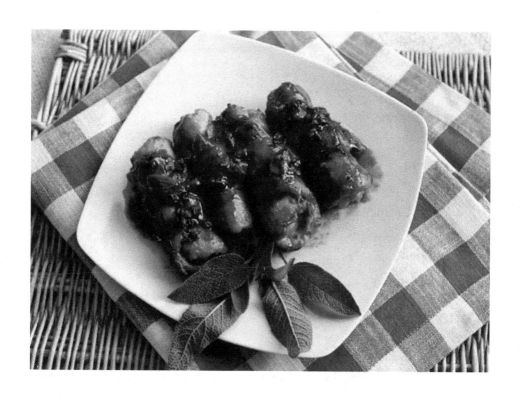

44. **Ham and Cheese Rollups**

Preparation Time: 5 minutes

Cooking Time: 8 minutes

Servings: 12

INGREDIENTS

- 2 tsp. raw honey
- 2 tsp. dried parsley
- 1 tbsp. poppy seeds
- ½ C. melted coconut oil
- ¼ C. spicy brown mustard
- 9 slices of provolone cheese
- 10 ounces of thinly sliced Black Forest Ham
- 1 tube of crescent rolls

DIRECTIONS

1. Roll out dough into a rectangle. Spread 2-3 tablespoons of spicy mustard onto dough, then layer provolone cheese and ham slices.
2. Roll the filled dough up as tight as you can and slice into 12-15 pieces.
3. Melt coconut oil and mix with a pinch of salt and pepper, parsley, honey, and remaining mustard.
4. Brush mustard mixture over roll-ups and sprinkle with poppy seeds.
5. Grease air fryer basket liberally with olive oil and add rollups.
6. Set temperature to 350°F, and set time to 8 minutes.

NUTRITIONS: Calories: 289 Fat: 6G Protein: 18G

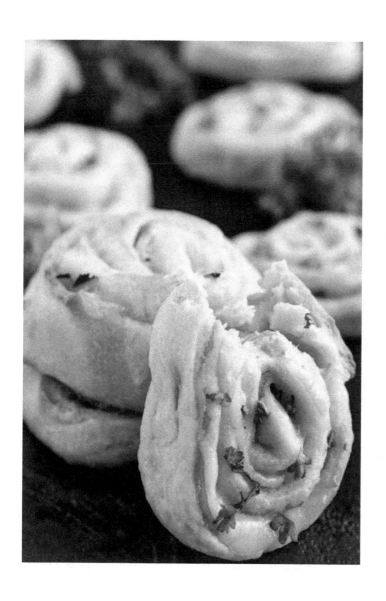

45. Vietnamese Pork Chops

Preparation Time: 10 minutes

Cooking Time: 7 minutes

Servings: 6

INGREDIENTS

- 1 tbsp. olive oil
- 1 tbsp. fish sauce
- 1 tsp. low-sodium dark soy sauce
- 1 tsp. pepper
- 3 tbsp. lemongrass
- 1 tbsp. chopped shallot
- 1 tbsp. chopped garlic
- 1 tbsp. brown sugar
- 2 pork chops

DIRECTIONS

1. Add pork chops to a bowl along with olive oil, fish sauce, soy sauce, pepper, lemongrass, shallot, garlic, and brown sugar.
2. Marinade pork chops 2 hours.
3. Ensure your air fryer is preheated to 400 degrees. Add pork chops to the basket.
4. Pour into the Oven rack/basket. Place the Rack on the middle-shelf of the Cosori Air Fryer Oven. Set temperature to 400°F, and set time to 7 minutes. Cook making sure to flip after 5 minutes of cooking.
5. Serve alongside steamed cauliflower rice.

NUTRITIONS: Calories: 290 Fat: 15G Protein: 30G Sugar: 3G

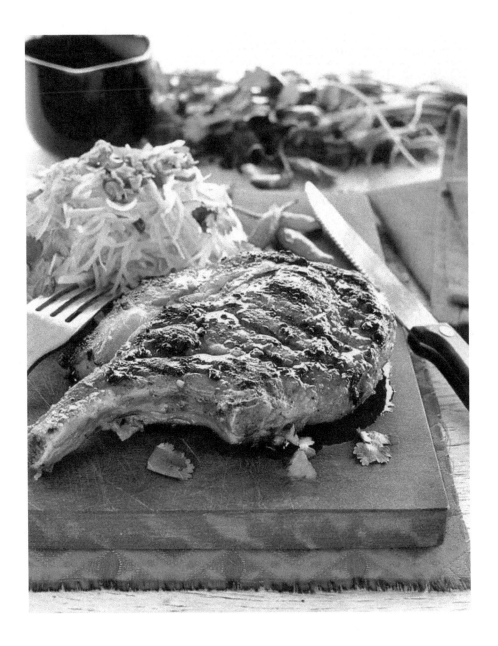

46. Basil Pork Chops

Preparation Time: 30 minutes

Cooking Time: 25 minutes

Servings: 4

INGREDIENTS

- 4 pork chops
- 2 tsp. basil; dried
- ½ tsp. chili powder
- 2 tbsp. olive oil
- A pinch of salt and black pepper

DIRECTIONS

1. In a pan that fits your air fryer, mix all the ingredients, toss.
2. Introduce in the fryer and cook at 400°F for 25 minutes. Divide everything between plates and serve

NUTRITION: Calories: 274 Fat: 13gFiber: 4g Carbs: 6g Protein: 18g

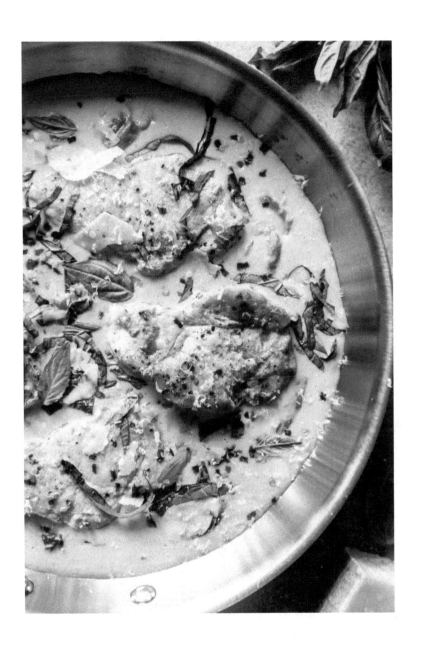

47. **Pub Burger**

Preparation Time: 20 minutes

Cooking Time: 10 minutes

Servings: 4

INGREDIENTS

- 8 large leaves butter lettuce
- 1 lb. ground sirloin
- 4 Bacon-Wrapped Onion Rings
- ½ cup full-fat mayonnaise
- 8 slices pickle
- 2 tbsp. salted butter; melted.
- 2 tsp. sriracha
- ¼ tsp. garlic powder.
- ½ tsp. salt
- ¼ tsp. ground black pepper

DIRECTIONS

1. Take a medium bowl, combine ground sirloin, salt and pepper. Form four patties. Brush each with butter and then place into the air fryer basket. Adjust the temperature to 380 Degrees F and set the timer for 10 minutes

2. Flip the patties halfway through the cooking time for a medium burger. Add an additional 3–5 minutes for well-done

3. In a small bowl, mix mayonnaise, sriracha and garlic powder. Set aside.

4. Place each cooked burger on a lettuce leaf and top with onion ring, two pickles and dollop of your prepared burger sauce. Wrap another lettuce leaf around tightly to hold. Serve warm.

NUTRITIONS: Calories: 442 Protein: 22.3g Fiber: 0.8g Fat: 34.9g Carbs: 4.1g

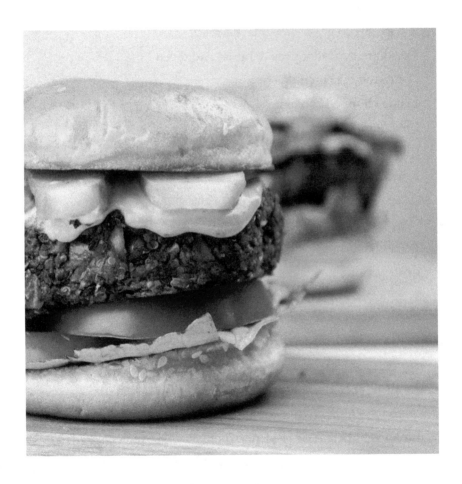

48. Pork Chop Salad

Preparation Time: 23 minutes

Cooking Time: 8 minutes

Servings: 2

INGREDIENTS

- 2, 4-oz.pork chops; chopped into 1-inch cubes
- ½ cup shredded Monterey jack cheese
- 1 medium avocado; peeled, pitted and diced
- ¼ cup full-fat ranch dressing
- 4 cups chopped romaine
- 1 medium Roma tomato; diced
- 1 tbsp. chopped cilantro
- 1 tbsp. coconut oil
- ½ tsp. garlic powder.
- ¼ tsp. onion powder.
- 2 tsp. chili powder
- 1 tsp. paprika

DIRECTIONS

1. Take a large bowl, drizzle coconut oil over pork. Sprinkle with chili powder, paprika, garlic powder and onion powder. Place pork into the air fryer basket.
2. Adjust the temperature to 400 Degrees F and set the timer for 8 minutes. Pork will be golden and crispy when fully cooked
3. Take a large bowl, place romaine, tomato and crispy pork. Top with shredded cheese and avocado. Pour ranch dressing around

bowl and toss the salad to evenly coat. Top with cilantro. Serve immediately.

NUTRITIONS: Calories: 526 Protein: 34.4g Fiber: 8.6g Fat: 37.0g Carbs: 13.8g

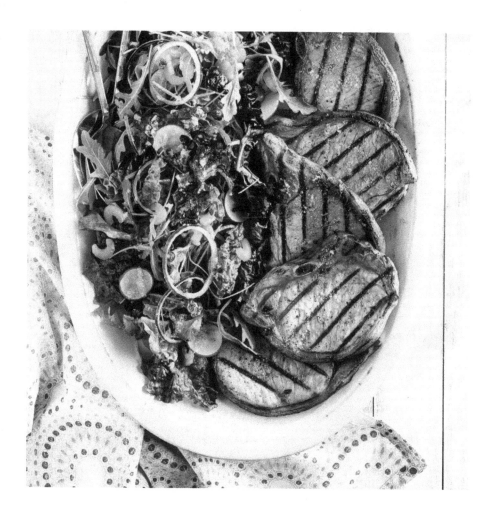

49. <u>Bacon Wrapped Hot Dog.</u>

Preparation Time: 15 minutes

Cooking Time: 10 minutes

Servings: 4

INGREDIENTS

- 4 slices sugar-free bacon.
- 4 beef hot dogs

DIRECTIONS

1. Wrap each hot dog with slice of bacon and secure with toothpick. Place into the air fryer basket.
2. Adjust the temperature to 370 Degrees F and set the timer for 10 minutes. Flip each hot dog halfway through the cooking time. When fully cooked, bacon will be crispy. Serve warm.

NUTRITIONS: Calories: 197 Protein: 9.2g Fiber: 0.0g Fat: 10g Carbs: 1.3g

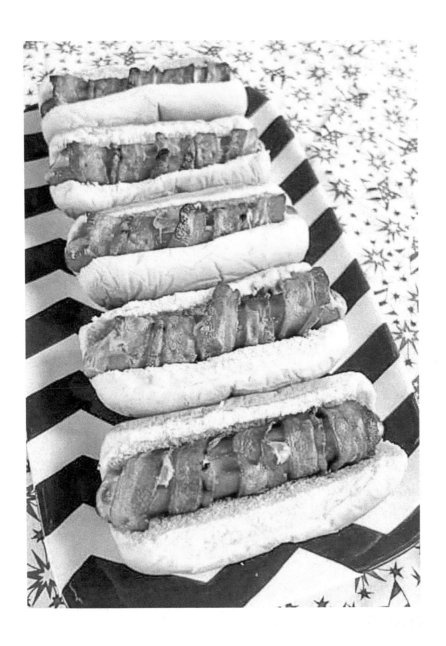

50. Easy Pork Chops

Preparation Time: 25 minutes

Cooking Time: 15 minutes

Servings: 4

INGREDIENTS

- 1½ oz. pork rinds, finely ground
- 1 tsp. chili powder
- ½ tsp. garlic powder.
- 1 tbsp. coconut oil; melted
- 4, 4-oz.pork chops

DIRECTIONS

1. Take a large bowl, mix ground pork rinds, chili powder and garlic powder.
2. Brush each pork chop with coconut oil and then press into the pork rind mixture, coating both sides. Place each coated pork chop into the air fryer basket
3. Adjust the temperature to 400 Degrees F and set the timer for 15 minutes. Flip each pork chop halfway through the cooking time
4. When fully cooked the pork chops will be golden on the outside and have an internal temperature of at least 145 Degrees F.

NUTRITIONS: Calories: 292 Protein: 29.5g Fiber: 0.3g Fat: 18.5g Carbs: 0.6g

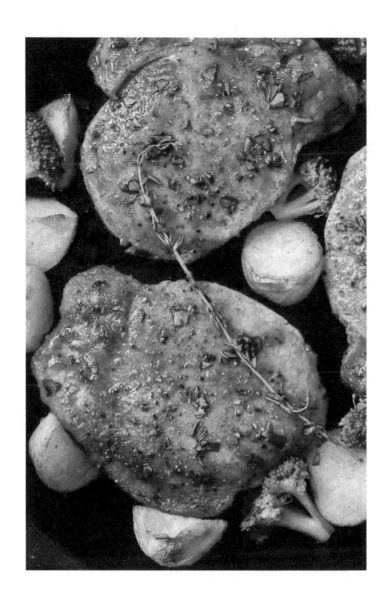

CONCLUSION

Now you know that Air fryer ovens are no less than a kitchen miracle, which have significantly brought ease and convenience with their user-friendly control systems, time and energy-efficient heating mechanism, and multiplicity of the cooking options. In this cookbook, the author has managed to share as many as different recipes, to provide an extensive guideline to all the frequent oven users. With its latest technology, you can bake, air fry, broil, dehydrate, toast, and roast all sorts of the meal, whether it is your morning breakfast or range of seafood, poultry, pork, beef, lamb, and vegetables. Give it a full read and find out tons of new ways to add more colors and flavors to your dinner table using the latest Air fryer ovens.

9 781803 400082